Empathetic Listening And Communication In Life, Love And Work

Dealing With Empathy Deficiencies Anywhere: Demonstrating Intentional Talk, Listening And Communication For Emotional Attunement

MOSES OMOJOLA

ISBN: **9798876882653**

DEDICATION

To the Glory of God.

CONTENTS

Introduction   1

1. Empathetic Communication Foundation   5

1.1: Understanding Life, Love, and Work Empathy   7

1.2: Empathy Deficits and Relationships   10

2. The Art of Intentional Talk   13

2.1: Meaningful Conversation crafting   15

2.2: Empathy Place in Difficult Discussions   18

3: Active Listening Power   23

3.1: Learning Active Listening   25

3.2: Overcoming Listening Barriers   29

4: Relationship Emotional Awareness   33

4.1: Connecting Emotionally   35

4.2: Attunement repairs and strengthens relationships   38

5. Empathetic Workplace Communication   43

5.1: Promoting Empathy   45

5.2: Professional Communication   49

6. Identifying and Correcting Empathy Deficits   55

6.1: Recognizing Empathy Deficits   55

6.2: Empathy Gap Strategies   57

7: Daily Empathetic Communication   63

7.1: Empathy in Daily Life   63

7.2: Long-Term Empathy Maintenance   66

Get Started Now!   75

ACKNOWLEDGMENTS

Special thanks to all those who contributed to the successful completion of this work.

Introduction

The book "Empathetic Listening and Communication in Life, Love, and Work: Dealing with Empathy Deficiencies Anywhere" covers deliberate conversation, empathetic listening, and emotional attunement. This book is a lighthouse for those who want to improve their interpersonal skills and make genuine relationships. The author understands the problems of empathy shortages in numerous facets of life.

Empathy, a fundamental human trait that frequently struggles in the fast-paced modern world, is the book's focus. The author uses significant study and practical experience to show how empathy helps people connect and navigate life, love, and work.

The book teaches readers how to listen empathetically, which is essential for meaningful interactions. It addresses the prevalent empathy deficits that can impair personal and professional interactions and offers solutions. Beyond theoretical talks, the book offers practical tasks to develop compassionate communication.

It centers on deliberate discourse, a thoughtful approach to interaction that bridges gaps. Readers should examine their communication habits, consider how their words affect others, and purposefully have discussions that foster understanding and connection.

The book's concepts apply to many situations due to its threefold focus on life, love, and work. Readers will learn how to improve their sympathetic communication abilities in family, personal, and professional relationships. Empathy, the author claims, is essential to success and happiness in all areas of life.

The book also encourages readers to uncover their compassionate qualities and growth areas. The author inspires people to actively participate in their relationships and fosters empathy and understanding in their personal and professional lives by taking a comprehensive approach to communication.

In an age of digital communication and fast-paced exchanges, "Empathetic Listening and Communication" helps reconnect with human connection.

1

Empathetic Communication Foundation

Foundation of Empathetic Communication examines the fundamentals of effective and compassionate communication. Recognizing and comprehending emotions, connecting, and creating trust underpin this notion. Healthy personal and professional relationships depend on compassionate communication.

To empathize with others, one must recognize and comprehend their feelings. Active listening, sensitivity, and genuine interest in the other person's perspective are needed. By noticing verbal and nonverbal clues, people may connect and affirm others' sentiments.

Empathetic communication relies on attentive listening. This requires listening, expressing interest, and giving comments that shows you understand their feelings. Active listening involves leaving aside one's own opinions and judgments to let the speaker speak freely. This technique fosters trust and openness, improving communication.

Empathetic communication requires emotional awareness and management. Sensitivity and empathy in talks require emotional intelligence.

Additionally, empathy requires seeing the world from another's perspective. Understanding others' unique experiences and feelings entails laying aside own prejudices and preconceptions. Empathy promotes inclusion and understanding in relationships by encouraging curiosity and openness to new ideas.

Another key of sympathetic communication is nonverbal communication. Expressions, gestures, and body language may convey emotions better than words. Understanding these nonverbal signs helps people empathize with others by revealing small changes in their emotional state.

Trust underpins compassionate communication. Trust requires constancy, honesty, and reliability. Trust grows when people feel heard and appreciated. Trust fosters free and honest conversation, making it safe to share sentiments.

1.1 UNDERSTANDING LIFE, LOVE, AND WORK EMPATHY

Our personal connections, work surroundings, and general well-being depend on empathy. It involves understanding and sharing others' sentiments, building relationships and support. Empathy underpins meaningful relationships and beneficial results in life, love, and business.

In interpersonal relationships, empathy underpins emotional connection. It involves thinking like another, feeling their feelings, and responding with empathy. This capacity fosters trust and closeness, enabling open conversation. Empathy develops links between people, helping them handle life's challenges together.

Love in all its manifestations feeds on empathy. Empathizing with one other's pleasures and sufferings strengthens love partnerships. This emotional attunement helps couples overcome obstacles, exhibit vulnerability, and grow closer. Love is an ongoing discourse of understanding, and empathy is its language.

Empathy boosts workplace cooperation and leadership. Building harmonious professional teams requires understanding colleagues' viewpoints and feelings. Empathetic leaders make workers feel seen, heard, and valued. This improves job happiness, productivity, and creativity. Empathy in the workplace builds resilience and inventiveness.

Empathy makes society healthier and more humane. It helps people respect various experiences and viewpoints, removing bias and misunderstanding. Empathy for persons of diverse races, cultures, and backgrounds promotes inclusion and social cohesiveness.

Empathy demands deliberate practice. It requires

active listening, nonjudgment, and presence. Self-empathy helps us understand and validate our feelings and show others kindness. Empathy requires persistent self-reflection and a dedication to understanding the human experience in all its complexity.

1.2 EMPATHY DEFICITS AND RELATIONSHIPS

Empathy deficits may badly damage relationships. Empathy inadequacies can emerge as an inability to grasp others' viewpoints, a lack of emotional reactivity, or disrespect for others' feelings.

Communication breaks broken due to empathy deficits. Partners might feel dissatisfied, resentful, and emotionally detached without empathy.

Empathy deficiencies may also diminish

relationships' emotional intimacy. Shared thoughts, feelings, and experiences foster closeness. One partner's lack of empathy may hinder a strong, lasting connection. People may struggle to provide emotional support and affirmation for meaningful relationships without empathy.

Empathy deficits can damage romantic trust. Trust is based on a partner understanding and respecting one's feelings and wants. Without empathy, couples may doubt one other's sincerity and intentions, losing trust. Insecurity, envy, and relational instability can result from this deterioration.

Empathy deficits affect friendships too. Over time, this imbalance might strain and terminate the connection. Teamwork and collaboration require empathy in the workplace.

2

The Art of Intentional Talk

The Art of Intentional Talk is a deep look at how intentional communication may build relationships, resolve issues, and achieve personal and professional success. In an age of instant communication, this helps people perfect their conversational abilities.

Intentional conversation is mindful communication. It goes beyond words to understanding, empathy, and genuineness. The book encourages readers to focus on their communication practices and go beyond surface-level interaction to more intentional participation.

Active listening is crucial here. Genuine communication includes listening and comprehending as much as speaking. Readers will learn how to improve their listening skills and connect with others.

Art of asking relevant questions is crucial. We discuss the importance of asking deep, thought-provoking questions. Readers must learn to question to get different ideas, find common ground, and negotiate various relationships.

Intentional communication in professional contexts will be examined alongside interpersonal interactions. Effective communication in leadership, teamwork, and negotiating is examined. We provide practical advice for executives who want to improve their communication skills, creating a more collaborative and inventive workplace.

In addition, intentions matters in conflict resolution. Instead of avoiding or intensifying disputes, we recommend thoughtful and purposeful conflict resolution. Emphasizing empathy, understanding, and open communication can help readers resolve issues constructively and build their relationships.

Readers are urged to evaluate their communication habits and find opportunities for development throughout this chapter. The author smoothly integrates research, real-life examples, and practical activities, making the book fascinating and useful to a wide audience.

2.1 MEANINGFUL CONVERSATION CRAFTING

Purposeful or intentional communication promotes

connection, understanding, and collaboration. Intentional talks in personal, professional, and educational settings can improve results and relationships. Consider these factors when talking intentionally.

It includes understanding the speaker's substance and emotion, not just hearing them. Make eye contact, nod, and confirm to show active listening. This respects the speaker and promotes free conversation.

Intentional communication should start with a defined aim or objective. If you're trying to understand a coworker, resolve a disagreement, or create rapport, a goal keeps the conversation on track. Set a focused and meaningful conversation by clearly stating your goals.

To stimulate deeper discussions, utilize open-ended questions that invite elaboration rather than one-word replies. These questions prompt thinking and emotional expression. Instead of "Did you enjoy the project?" ask, "What aspects of the project did you find most engaging, and why?"

Empathy and Understanding: Intentional communication entails emotional connection with people. Acknowledge and validate the speaker's emotions to show empathy. Learn their perspective, even if it varies from yours. This builds trust and respect, enabling deeper interactions.

Mindful Communication: Intentional communication requires mindfulness. Be sensitive to nonverbal clues and avoid interrupting. Communication is more genuine and effective when present. To have a healthy and productive conversation, you must recognize and manage your emotions.

Feedback and Reflection: Intentional communication is mutual. Encourage participant input to ensure everyone is heard and understood. Reflect on the conversation to find insights and ways to improve. Reflection increases deliberate conversation learning and progress.

In different situations, cultural awareness is essential for effective communication. Consider cultural differences and respect others' opinions when talking. This prevents misconceptions and fosters a more diverse conversation.

Flexibility and adaptability are essential for effective purposeful communication. Be flexible with your communication style to suit the participants. Flexibility makes conversations more dynamic and responsive, allowing everyone to speak.

2.2 EMPATHY PLACE IN DIFFICULT DISCUSSIONS

Empathy is essential for understanding and resolving challenging conversations. Empathy may improve personal, business, and social discussions. Remember these fundamentals:

1. Actively Listen: Start by hearing the other person out. Give them your entire attention and don't interrupt or plan your response. Nodding, establishing eye contact, and paraphrasing to clarify shows you appreciate their opinion. This fosters mutual respect.

2. Validate Emotions: Accept the other party's feelings.

3. Communicate Your Feelings: Share your thoughts and feelings without conflict. Use "I" expressions to prevent accusation. Try "I feel concerned when..." This technique encourages open communication and helps others understand your perspective without feeling attacked.

4. Find Common Ground: Find common ground with the other person. Finding answers might start with common beliefs or aims. Before discussing disagreements, emphasize your similarities. This can minimize stress and boost collaboration.

5. Reduce Blame and Accusations: Instead of blaming the other person, stress shared responsibility. Blaming escalates tension and makes

the other person defensive. Say "I think we both have a role to play in finding a solution" instead than "This is all your fault."

6. Be Open to Change: Be ready to change your mind during the talk. This doesn't imply compromising your values, but it does require accepting new ideas. Allowing change creates an environment where both sides can learn.

7. Say "We": Use inclusive language like "we" when discussing solutions or next actions to show teamwork. This changes the dialog from combative to cooperative.

8. When to Take a Break: If emotions are high and the talk is unproductive, offer a break. Taking a break lets both sides calm down and reflect. You

can avoid an argument by doing this.

3

Active Listening Power

Communication affects how we interact, form connections, and manage our personal and professional life. Active listening is one of the most transforming communication abilities. Active listening fosters comprehension, empathy, and meaningful relationships by deeply engaging with the speaker.

Active hearing goes beyond passive receiving. It is dynamic and involves purposeful effort and a real desire to understand the message. Today's fast-paced environment, when distractions abound and true connection is sometimes overlooked, makes this ability vital. By practicing active listening, people may reap several advantages beyond the discourse.

Active listening requires setting aside one's own ideas and judgments to properly absorb the speaker's message. Hearing the words and comprehending their emotions, intents, and subtleties is necessary. Trust and rapport are built when people feel heard and understood. This fosters good personal and professional connections. Active listening helps develop and sustain successful partnerships in a world where collaboration and teamwork are crucial.

By understanding others' opinions and concerns, people may make educated decisions that consider several perspectives. This collaborative approach improves results and promotes inclusion and respect.

Conflict resolution is another important part of active listening. Every human contact involves misunderstandings and conflicts, yet attentively listening may reduce tensions and discover common ground. The empathy that comes with active listening helps individuals resolve problems and progress through compromise.

Actively listening leaders show empathy, transparency, and genuine concern for their team members. This improves morale and workplace collaboration.

3.1 LEARNING ACTIVE LISTENING

Effective communication and comprehension need active listening. Hearing words is not enough—you must concentrate, comprehend, respond, and remember them.

Here are some essential active listening techniques:

1. Give Full Attention: Active listening requires full attention to the speaker. Avoid distractions, put aside electronics, and look at each other. Showing you're present shows the speaker you value their message.

2. Demonstrate Active Listening: Non-verbal signals are effective clues. Nodding, welcoming stance, and engaging facial expressions show attention. Avoid fidgeting and checking your phone, which indicate boredom.

3. Paraphrase and Reflect: Reflect on the speaker's

message to guarantee comprehension. This shows you understand and lets the speaker elaborate.

4. Ask Clarifying Questions: This shows your interest and guarantees you understand. Open-ended queries prompt further information.

5. Give Feedback: Your feedback shows that you are actively listening and digesting the material.

6. Avoid Interrupting: Avoid interrupting or completing the speaker's statements. Allow them to finish before answering. Interrupting might make the speaker feel unheard and interrupt the discourse. Patience is essential to active listening.

7.   Foster   Empathy: Active   listening   entails comprehending both words and feelings. Think like the speaker and feel their emotions. Empathy builds trust and connection in communication.

8. Practice Mindfulness: Being present in the moment may greatly improve active listening. Mindful listening improves comprehension and connection.

9. Maintain a cheerful Attitude: Be open and cheerful in all conversations. Positive thinking improves communication and idea sharing. Be engaged in the speaker's message to improve your active listening.

10. Commit to Continuous Improvement: Active

listening, like any ability, can be optimized with time. Ask for feedback, evaluate your encounters, and improve. You may improve your communication skills and empathy by continuing your growth.

3.2 OVERCOMING LISTENING BARRIERS

Building connections, improving communication, and developing personally and professionally requires overcoming listening hurdles.

2. Eliminate Distractions: Environmental and physical distractions might hamper listening.

3. Maintain Eye Contact: This nonverbal indication

boosts confidence and encourages open conversation.

4. Maintain Open-Mind: Engage in talks without previous beliefs or biases. Be open to fresh ideas and don't assume the speaker's stance.

5. Empathy and Understanding: Put yourself in the speaker's shoes to develop empathy. This emotional bond supports communication.

6. Paraphrase and Summarize: Practice these skills to accurately grasp the speaker's message. This shows you comprehend and shows the speaker you appreciate their message.

7. Manage Internal Monologue: Internal distractions like replies or self-criticism might hinder effective listening. Be alert and return to the speaker when these distractions occur.

8. Cultural Sensitivity: Appreciate and understand diverse communication approaches. Cultural differences in language, subtleties, and nonverbal clues should be considered.

9. Seek input: Ask people for input on your listening abilities. This might help you identify areas for development and strengthen your communication.

10. Patience and Tolerance: Be patient while handling difficult or emotive matters. Give the

speaker time to talk without judging.

11. Be Mentally Present: Focus on talks. Stop multitasking and thinking about other things while listening. Being totally present helps you understand the talk.

12. Continuous Learning: Seek chances to enhance your listening abilities. Attend workshops, read books, or take communication and listening courses.

13. Establish a feedback loop with the speaker to guarantee mutual comprehension. Encourage them to comment on how well you understood their message and if any clarification is required.

4

Relationship Emotional Awareness

In partnerships, emotional attunement helps people comprehend and connect with their partners' feelings, fostering empathy.

Emotionally attuned partners notice verbal and nonverbal clues and show genuine interest in one other. This provides emotional security and helps people feel heard and understood.

Communication is essential for emotional awareness. To create vulnerability and connection, partners must disclose their feelings and opinions.

Communicating effectively requires sharing pleasant feelings and handling disagreements and challenges with empathy and understanding. This procedure enhances emotional closeness and relationship bonding.

Attunement to emotions requires empathy. Empathetic reactions strengthen and validate relationships.

Additionally, emotional attunement requires emotional management. Partners must control their emotions to establish a stable emotional environment. This entails identifying and managing emotional reactions, keeping disagreements from escalating, and establishing relationship emotional equilibrium. Emotion control improves partnership harmony and resilience.

Successful emotional attunement requires emotional intelligence. This requires self-awareness and knowledge of others' feelings. Emotional intelligence helps people manage interpersonal dynamics and improve communication and connection.

4.1 CONNECTING EMOTIONALLY

Personal and professional interactions require emotional connection. You can build strong emotional relationships through these:

1. Active Listening: Stop interrupting and show you understand.

2. Empathy: The capacity to comprehend and experience the emotions of another person. Take their place, respect their feelings, and affirm their

experiences. Hearing and being understood deepens emotional connections.

3. Encourage Open Communication: Set up an environment that promotes open communication. Be open about your feelings. This vulnerability makes others feel comfortable doing the same, building a real relationship.

4. Shared Experiences: Participate in memorable events. Shared hobbies, travel, or simply a simple dinner provide a sense of closeness and emotional connection.

5. Express thanks: Regularly show thanks to those in your life. Let them know you appreciate their efforts and presence. Feeling gratitude enhances

relationships.

6. Support in Tough Times: Emotional ties need being there for people throughout difficult times. Be supportive, listen, and encourage. Standing by someone in need strengthens the emotional bond.

7. Celebrate Successes: Recognize and honor others' accomplishments. Sharing successes boosts mood and connection. Recognizing one other's successes strengthens relationships.

8. Reading nonverbal cues

Be aware to body language and facial emotions. Often, small cues convey feelings. Be aware of these indications to respond correctly and build the emotional connection.

9. Respect diversity: Appreciating and valuing individual diversity is essential for emotional bonds. Admire and respect variations in idea, opinion, and viewpoint.

10. Time and Consistency: Emotional relationships need sustained work. Spend time with your connections through excellent talks, shared activities, or just being together. Trust and emotional relationships are strengthened by consistency.

4.2 ATTUNEMENT REPAIRS AND STRENGTHENS RELATIONSHIPS

Attunement is a wonderful technique to reconnect with people. Tuning into others' emotions and needs fosters understanding and connection.

Here are some effective attunement methods to mend and improve relationships:

1. Active Listening: Attunement relies on active listening. Put aside distractions, look at people, and don't interrupt. Restate what you hear to demonstrate your understanding. You acknowledge their sentiments and show your devotion to the connection.

2. Empathy: Accept their feelings and sympathize. This fosters trust and closeness.

3. Open Communication: Promote honest communication. Create a secure area for both sides to express their feelings without judgment. Share your feelings and experiences too. Trust and emotional bonding increase with transparency.

4. Non-Verbal Cues: Observe body language and facial emotions. These indicators frequently tell more about a person's feelings than words. Respond to these indications to demonstrate your awareness of their requirements.

Step 5: Validate the other person's feelings and experiences. Accept their feelings and show you understand. Validation fosters acceptance and affirmation, which is crucial for relationship restoration.

6. Apologize and Forgive: Apologize for misunderstandings or disagreements where you contributed. Being accountable shows maturity and dedication to the partnership. Keeping grudges might impair attunement.

7. Quality Time: Enhance emotional connection via quality time together. Make memories by doing something you both like. Sharing experiences unites and strengthens relationships.

8. Constancy: Attunement demands continuing constancy. Maintain active listening, empathy, and open communication in your relationship. Consistency strengthens trust and emotional bonds.

5

Empathetic Workplace Communication

Empathetic workplace communication promotes strong connections, cooperation, and a healthy, inclusive workplace. Understanding others' thoughts and viewpoints, encouraging open discourse, and building team trust are key to this communication approach. Today's diverse workplaces require empathy, which boosts employee well-being and business performance.

Empathetic communication requires attentive listening. This requires focusing, comprehending, reacting, and remembering what others say. Genuine attention and focus may make coworkers feel valued and understood. This may boost teamwork, eliminate misunderstandings, and strengthen bonds.

Conflict resolution also requires empathy. Understanding the feelings and concerns of all sides in workplace disagreements is crucial to developing lasting solutions. Empathetic communication encourages people to examine the emotions and motives behind opposing views rather than just the facts. This strategy encourages compassion and cooperation, helping teams overcome problems.

Empathy aids leadership and conflict resolution. Empathetic leaders are more aware of team needs. Instilling trust and loyalty in employees through understanding and support boosts morale and productivity. This leadership style promotes an inclusive, collaborative workplace where varied opinions are appreciated and everyone is heard.

Creating a corporate culture of empathy needs conscious efforts to make people feel secure sharing their feelings. Open communication, openness, and discouraging judgment are needed. Team-building, training, and check-ins may foster empathy.

Organizations must realize how empathic communication affects employee well-being and work satisfaction. Empathy-focused organizations have fewer stress, burnout, and attrition, according to research. Empathetic workplaces motivate, engage, and commit employees. This boosts individual and organizational achievement.

In conclusion, empathic communication fosters great workplace connections and a strong culture.

5.1 PROMOTING EMPATHY

Creating a friendly workplace requires promoting empathy. When employees feel understood and respected, they cooperate better, speak more openly, and help the company succeed. Here are some workplace empathy strategies:

1. Lead by Example: Empathy cultivation begins at the top. Leaders should show staff empathy. Leaders who listen, understand, and care establish a great tone for the organization.

2. Foster Open Communication: Encourage employees to voice their opinions and feelings. Regular team meetings, feedback channels, and openness promote open communication. People show greater empathy when they feel heard.

3. Workshops and Trainings: Do these to promote workplace empathy, training can be continuous.

4. Recognize and Celebrate Diversity: Promote a culture of diversity rather than judgment. People feel respected and understood in an inclusive workplace.

5. Flexible Work Arrangements: Offer flexible work arrangements to address varied employee demands and difficulties. Flexibility shows understanding for team members' individual requirements.

6. Recognize and Appreciate Employees: Team recognition promotes morale and shows that the

company values them. Simple thanks may create a happy and sympathetic workplace.

7. Implement supportive policies to promote work-life balance, mental health, and general well-being. When workers perceive their company values their health and happiness, empathy and loyalty grow.

8. Team-Building events: Organize events that foster collaboration and connection among team members.

Promote Empathetic Leadership: Give leaders and managers the means to lead with empathy. Leadership that addresses employee needs promotes empathy throughout the company.

10. Feedback and Continuous Improvement: Create a feedback loop for employee input on workplace culture. Create constant employee experience enhancements using this feedback. Empathy is strengthened when employees' views are heard and improvements are done.

5.2 PROFESSIONAL COMMUNICATION

Effective professional communication is essential for a happy workplace, healthy connections, and organizational success. Here are some workplace communication tips:

1. Effective communication relies heavily on active listening. Listen carefully, ask questions, and repeat crucial topics to ensure you understand. Avoid

interrupting and focus on the speaker to show respect and comprehension.

Use clear and succinct communication to convey your ideas. Jargon and complex words might confuse your viewers. Use clear, concise language and arrange your thoughts to communicate.

3. Select the Right Medium: Choose the right communication channel for your message. Face-to-face contact is best for sensitive or difficult issues, although email may be better for specific information. Know each communication medium's pros and cons and pick accordingly.

4. Be Aware of Non-Verbal Cues: Body language and facial expressions significantly impact

communication. Be attentive of your own and others' nonverbal cues. To project confidence and sincerity, make eye contact, utilize open body language, and watch your tone.

5. Target Your Audience: The Communication style changes improve comprehension and engagement.

6. Give Constructive Feedback: Focus on particular actions or outcomes and provide constructive feedback, not criticism. Feedback should inspire improvement and suggest answers or alternatives. Keep good contributions in mind for balanced communication.

7. Communicate Expectations: Clarify expectations to prevent confusion. Make sure everyone knows

their position and the expected results whether assigning tasks, creating objectives, or delegating duties. Check for alignment and correct issues regularly.

8. Building Emotional Intelligence: Improve emotional intelligence for successful interpersonal connections. Be mindful of your own and others' emotions and how they affect communication. Empathy and understanding foster teamwork.

9. Be Open to Feedback: Encourage open communication by staying open to feedback. Encourage coworkers to voice issues and aggressively seek feedback. Feedback improves work relationships and continual progress.

10. Professional Etiquette: Show professionalism in every conversation. Use polite language, avoid gossip, and respect people. Consider your team's diversity and workplace culture.

6

Identifying and Correcting Empathy Deficits

There is need to show how empathy deficits affect individuals and society. People without empathy may have trouble communicating, developing relationships, and navigating complicated social dynamics. Empathy deficiencies can erode community compassion, which may raise disputes and lower communal well-being.

To discover empathy weaknesses, look for signs including difficulties recognizing and comprehending others' feelings, emotional insensitivity, and perspective-taking issues. To enhance their conduct and relationships, people must be self-aware.

We wish to discuss realistic empathy-building methods. Active listening requires focusing, comprehending, reacting, and remembering what others say. These talents improve emotional connection and comprehension of other views.

Mindfulness is also advised. Mindfulness is being present, acknowledging one's feelings, and being aware of others'. Mindfulness can help people understand their emotions and those of others.

Education promotes empathy, too. The necessity of educating children how to recognize and manage emotions is stressed in its call for empathy-building programs in schools and workplaces. Such programs can help develop empathic, socially capable people who can build healthy relationships.

We recommend using technology to boost empathy. VR and internet platforms may imitate real-world circumstances, allowing people to exercise empathy in a controlled context. These technologies can help folks who struggle with face-to-face encounters practice and improve their empathy abilities in a secure environment.

6.1 RECOGNIZING EMPATHY DEFICITS

Interactions require empathy to build understanding, connection, and collaboration. Some people have low empathy. Recognizing empathy deficits can help personal growth and relationships. Watch for these signs:

1. Inadequate Emotional Response: Lack of

empathy might hinder individuals from responding correctly to others' feelings. They may ignore delight, grief, or irritation.

2. Challenging Meaningful Connections: They may feel alone or have trouble maintaining friendships and love relationships due to their inability to develop intimate attachments.

3. Limited Non-Verbal Cues: Facial expressions, body language, and tone of voice heavily impact communication and empathy. These indicators may be misinterpreted by those with empathy deficits, causing miscommunication and a lack of connection.

4. Support Difficulties: Empathy requires both

understanding and offering support for others' feelings. Empathy-deficient people may struggle to console, encourage, or help during difficult times. Cold or aloof replies make it hard for others to seek help from them.

6.2 EMPATHY GAP STRATEGIES

Beyond personal connections, empathy deficits can affect professional encounters. These gaps emerge when people struggle to relate to another' feelings and experiences. Empathy bridges are essential for building deeper relationships and a more compassionate and inclusive society. Several methods can help bridge empathy gaps:

1. One key to bridging empathy gaps is active listening. Give your undivided attention to the

speaker, prevent interruptions, and attempt to grasp their perspective. Validating the other person's feelings and reflecting on their words might help bridge the gap.

2. Adopt a perspective-taking approach: Explore the world from someone else's perspective. They must imagine their ideas, feelings, and experiences without judgment. Perspective-taking helps develop empathy by helping you comprehend their feelings and behaviors.

3. Self-Education: Lack of information or awareness of specific situations might lead to empathy gaps. Read books, watch documentaries, and talk to varied individuals to increase empathy.

4. Develop Emotional Intelligence: Recognize and comprehend your own and others' emotions. Mastering this ability helps you bridge empathy barriers. Body language and facial expressions may reveal someone's feelings.

5. Foster Open Communication: Establish a culture of value for honest communication. Encourage others to speak freely without judgment. This reduces obstacles and promotes genuine communication and understanding.

6. Practice empathy activities to improve emotional connections with people. Role-playing, empathy seminars, and mindfulness can help you understand your own and others' emotions.

7. Seek input: Constantly seek outside input on your empathy skills. Ask how you might better understand and help them. Constructive comments can help you bridge empathy gaps.

8. Reflect on your prejudices, assumptions, and preconceptions regularly. Think about how these elements affect your empathy. Being conscious of your limitations helps you overcome them and be more open-minded.

9. Lead by Example: Exhibit empathy in your dealings. Witnessing empathy might motivate others to develop it. Be a personal and professional exemplar of empathy.

7

Daily Empathetic Communication

Empathetic communication improves relationships, understanding, and society.

Active listening - Concentrating, comprehending, reacting, and remembering what is spoken is required. By listening without interrupting or condemning, we provide a safe environment for the speaker to talk. Active listening helps us connect with people and shows our interest in their perspectives.

Empathetic communication requires attentive

listening and nonverbal signals. Facial expressions, body language, and eye contact show real attention and care. Being aware of our nonverbal clues helps us communicate openly. Even when words fail, a look or touch may show empathy.

Using words to show empathy is crucial. Validating someone's sentiments creates understanding and support. Avoid making assumptions or proposing answers too fast, as this can damage empathy.

Self-awareness is key to regular compassionate conversation. Understanding our emotions helps us empathize with others. Reflecting on our own experiences and how they connect to others' helps us comprehend. Self-awareness helps us control our emotions, reducing disputes and improving relationships.

Empathy is caring and helping, not just understanding emotions. No matter how tiny, acts of kindness increase empathy. These actions of listening, helping, or showing concern foster empathy in our daily lives.

To foster empathy, one must be open to variety and other viewpoints. Accepting the diversity of human experiences and opinions helps us connect with others. We make society more inclusive and empathic by actively seeking varied ideas and having polite talks.

7.1 Empathy in Daily Life

Empathy in daily encounters strengthens relationships, builds connections, and positively impacts others. Daily life may be lived with empathy, which entails understanding and sharing others' feelings.

Here are some methods to use empathy in daily life:

1. Active Listening: Empathy relies heavily on active listening. Listen intently without interrupting or planning your response. Show your interest in the discourse by nodding, making eye contact, and speaking. This clarifies their perspective and makes them feel heard and respected.

2. Consider their perspective: Visualize the world from their perspective. Consider their sentiments, experiences, and situations. This doesn't imply you have to agree, but knowing their position builds rapport. Consider how you would feel in their circumstance and respond accordingly.

3. offer Understanding: After listening and acknowledging the other person's feelings or

experiences, offer your understanding. Use words like "I can see how that would be challenging" a "I understand why you feel that way." This shows you understand and acknowledges their feelings.

4. Avoid Judgments: Empathy demands an open mind. Avoid hasty conclusions about others. Judgement might hamper your capacity to connect with others because everyone has different experiences and struggles. Instead, be curious and open-minded.

5. Validate feelings: Acknowledge the feelings of others. Validation implies acknowledging their sentiments, not agreeing. I can comprehend "It's okay to feel that way" and "I can see why you might feel that way".

6. Provide assistance: During difficult times, provide assistance. This might be as basic as showing sympathy or aiding them. Be there for them and offer any help you can. Actions frequently trump words.

7. Consider Non-Verbal Cues: Be aware of such indicators to interpret the words' sentiments. A soothing touch or smile may show empathy without words.

8. Practice Patience: Empathy takes time and patience. Avoid rushing the topic and let others speak. Patience shows you understand and support others.

7.2 LONG-TERM EMPATHY MAINTENANCE

Empathy is essential for productive interactions and self-care in a fast-paced, demanding society. Long-term empathy takes intentionality and attention.

For lifelong well-being, try these ways to keep empathy at the center of your life.

1. Develop Self-Compassion:

Empathy begins inward. To maintain empathy, practice self-compassion. Kindly accept your challenges and treat yourself with the same empathy you show others. Maintaining a positive self-image helps you sympathize with others.

2. Set Limits:

Establishing appropriate boundaries is as crucial as empathy. Exhaustion from overwork might result. Be aggressive in setting boundaries and knowing your limits. This isn't about denying empathy, but rather having the energy and emotional resources to sustain it.

3. Actively Listen:

Understanding and active listening build empathy. Try to focus on talks and prevent distractions. Doing so improves your empathy and bonds with others.

4. Develop Supportive Networks:

Find people who value and reciprocate empathy. Having a supporting network might help maintain empathy. Sharing stories, seeking advice, and offering support in this group creates a positive feedback loop that fosters empathy.

5. Reflect often.

Review your sympathetic experiences often. Consider how your empathy helped and find areas for improvement. Reflection improves self-awareness and compassionate skills.

6. Learn constantly:

Experience and knowledge develop empathy. Be open to other cultures, ideas, and viewpoints. Learn constantly to comprehend others' different experiences. This progress will increase your empathy and well-being.

7. Practice mindfulness:

Mindfulness improves empathy by keeping you present. Practicing meditation, deep breathing, or other mindfulness techniques can help you stay aware of your own and others' emotions.

8. Honor Empathetic Success:

Honor your empathic efforts that have helped others. Recognize the delight and fulfillment of profound emotional connections. Celebrating these accomplishments reinforces empathy in your life.

Get Started Now!

In the last chapters of "Empathetic Listening And Communication In Life, Love And Work," profound insight and revolutionary action meet. After studying empathy and its importance in personal and professional relationships, it is obvious that empathy deficits can prevent true connection. With this exploration's findings, we may overcome these barriers and promote conscious conversation, deep listening, and empathic communication.

These pages have guided you through human

connection's intricacies. We've examined empathy's components to understand how it unites people in life, love, and work. We've faced empathy deficits, which may destroy relationships without purposeful effort.

Knowing this, we must deliberately display intentional conversation, listening, and communication for emotional attunement. We have power in our daily encounters at home, work, and in the community. It's about seeing every discussion as a chance to build empathy.

Let's be empathetic listeners who comfort people and communicators who inspire them. Let us be partners who understand without judgment, confidants who share weaknesses, and sensitive hearts that build unbreakable relationships in love. Let us be diverse-minded coworkers, empathetic leaders, and harmonious team members at work.

Communication must be purposeful to address empathy deficits. It requires developing empathy as a talent, art, and lifestyle. Let this chapter conclude with an invitation to embrace the transforming power of empathic listening and communication, which may break down boundaries, create understanding, and build bridges across human connection.

May our deliberate actions stitch empathy, understanding, and steadfast connection into our lives.

ABOUT THE AUTHOR

I am the author of that famous book: "How to discover your divine destiny and total breakthroughs". I spent 16 years working as an Engineer in the Oil and Gas industry before I was divinely conscripted into my divine assignment. I am an author, international speaker, counselor, destiny mentor, business and wellness coach. My specialties are hidden truths, divine assignment, justice, success and leadership.

I run workshops to help people discover their destiny, the unique business God created them to do, how to start and succeed. I also counsel individuals empathetically on issues relating to destiny, employment, health, relationships, and many more, using the awesome power inherent in their destiny, and assist many to become writers and self – publish many books.

www.ingramcontent.com/pod-product-compliance
Lightning Source LLC
Chambersburg PA
CBHW060957260726
48661CB00005B/1917